INTERMITTENT FASTING FOR WOMEN OVER 50

A SIMPLE AND HEALTHY WAY TO TAKE CONTROL OF YOUR BODY; LOSE WEIGHT, INCREASE YOUR ENERGY, DELAY AGING, AND FEEL GREAT

TABLE OF CONTENTS

INTRODUCTION

What is Intermittent Fasting?

Intermittent fasting is a technique that extends the time of each day you are not eating, whether you're skipping breakfast to get a head start on dinner or not eating lunch so you can have an extended break at work. This increases the amount of time your body uses fat for energy and helps break the constant eating cycle, so you don't feel hungry. This means that you go longer between meals before eating again while maintaining your weight and making fat loss easier. This is done by counting 24 hours out of every day and fasting for 8-16 hours from most food sources (the fast time can be a little more or less than eight hours, such as 10 or 12). This will work best if done within a 16-hour feeding window where all meals are nutritious and low in refined carbs and sugars.

If this sounds familiar, then it's probably because you have heard about intermittent fasting before.

How Does Intermittent Fasting Work?

Rather than consuming your calories over a few hours, intermittent fasting brings them together into one meal. This means that doing your normal four hours daily fast and then breaking it up over 12 hours would require six meals (three times per day). However, if you spend more time between eating (say 24 hours), it would mean just one meal for those 24 hours.

How Can Intermittent Fasting Help You Lose Weight?

Intermittent fasting helps with weight loss by allowing your body to do more of the work for you.

When you eat a large meal, your body uses the glucose in the blood for energy. The glucose is then stored in the liver and muscles as glycogen, so it will always be there if needed. When you are fasting, your body has to use what is stored, and it starts to burn fat instead of sugar. This means that your body will start to use up excess fat that much quicker and help you achieve your weight loss goals without spending long hours at the gym.

The science behind Intermittent Fasting

Intermittent fasting is a great way to lose weight and become healthier because your body is forced to rely on its fat stores for power. This means that you draw off currently stored fats rather than increase your intake of fats and carbohydrates. When you introduce intermittent fasting into your weight loss plan, you will become healthier while still losing those stubborn pounds.

How Intermittent Fasting Helps Women Over 50

In general, women tend to have more fat in their bodies than men, but this doesn't mean they can't fit into their dream dresses or even look good in a two-piece bathing suit. Here are some points on how intermittent fasting helps women over 50:

1. Allows to lose weight
2. Helps to improve blood sugar levels
3. It's easy to follow, especially for the busy woman over 50
4. It's something that can be done while still enjoying your favorite foods and drinks
5. Helps boost energy levels, and keeps you healthy and active throughout the day
6. It increases your lifespan

When you are over 50, your metabolism slows down compared to those younger, so it's harder to lose weight or maintain a decent weight level without spending a lot of time exercising and dieting. Intermittent fasting can give you the chance to eat like you normally do while still helping with your weight loss goals. Intermittent fasting increases the body's fat-burning capabilities by speeding up your metabolism, so it becomes easier for your body to burn through excess fat and weight.

Overall, intermittent fasting is a great way to keep fit and healthy while also helping you shed off those extra pounds.

How to Intermittent Fasting for Women Over 50?

When it comes to fasting, every diet book says, "You're too old for that." But recent research found out that women in their 50s can still fast and get some weight loss results.

Intermittent fasting is an absolutely natural process of the human body, where your body doesn't eat for a certain period, and when you eat again, you replenish all the lost energy. This is what our ancestors did to survive. Something we rarely do nowadays! A key component of intermittent fasting is 'not eating,' but rather taking meal breaks or limiting your eating hours.

So, let us begin your journey to your desired weight with the help of Intermittent Fasting!

CHAPTER 1: DIETS AND PSYCHOLOGICAL STRESS

Some individuals demonstrate mind-boggling protection from limits of temperature. Consider Buddhist priests who can tranquility withstand being hung in solidifying towels or the purported "Iceman" Wim Hof, who can stay submerged in ice water for significant periods without inconvenience.

These individuals will, in general, be seen as superhuman or exceptional somehow or another. If they are, at that point, their accomplishments are engaging yet superfluous vaudevillian acts. However, imagine a scenario in which they're not monstrosities yet have prepared their minds and bodies with self-change procedures that give them cold obstruction. Would anyone be able to do likewise?

As two neuroscientists who have considered how the human mind reacts to the introduction to cold, we are charmed by what occurs in the cerebrum during such opposition. Our exploration, and that of others, is starting to propose these sorts of "superpowers" may be a possible outcome from deliberately rehearsing methods that change one's cerebrum or body. These adjustments might be applicable for social and emotional well-being and can be tackled by anybody.

The Body's Drive for Balance

Social change procedures like yoga and care aim to balance physiological balance in what researchers call homeostasis. Homeostasis is an essential endurance need and critical for a creature's physical uprightness. For instance, when somebody is presented with the cold, certain mind focuses start to change how the body reacts. These incorporate diminishing the bloodstream to the limits and enacting profound layer muscle gatherings to create heat. These progressions let the body clutch a greater amount of its warmth and happen naturally without conscious control.

Homeostasis is kept up when fringe organs ("the body") gather tangible information and forward it to the preparing focus ("the cerebrum"), which composes and organizes this information, creating activity plans. These orders are then passed on to the body, which executes them.

The harmony between base-up physiological components and top-down mental instruments intercedes homeostasis and aides' activities. Our thought is that this harmony among physiology and brain science can be "hacked" via preparing the cerebrum to manage introduction to cold. This is an exceptionally intriguing stunt, and we accept the cerebrum changes that happen to reach out past simply cool resilience.

Mind Frameworks for Reacting to Cold

Mind frameworks for keeping up homeostasis structure a perplexing chain of importance. Anatomical areas in the crude brainstem (midbrain, pons) and the nerve center structure a homeostatic system. This system makes a portrayal of the body's present physiologic state.

Given what this portrayal depicts about the body's conditions, administrative procedures trigger physiological changes in the outskirts through the sensory system. The portrayal likewise produces essential passionate reactions to physiologic changes, "cold is upsetting", and those trigger activities "I have to get inside."

In people, a territory in the back of the midbrain called the periaqueductal dim is the control focus that sends messages about agony and cold to the body. This territory discharges narcotics and cannabinoids, mind synthetic concoctions likewise connected with a state of mind and nervousness. The periaqueductal dark sends these compound signs both to the body, through the slipping pathway that smothers the experience of agony and cold, and using different synapses to the mind.

Like those related to the cerebrum stem, lower-request crude systems developed before higher-request locales of the mind, similar to those in its cortex. Also, lower-request systems apply a more prominent effect on higher-request systems. Here's an unmistakable model: Being seriously cool will meddle with normal thinking, a condition that in hypothermia is disastrous. In any case, one can't just envision a radiant seashore to wash away the repulsiveness related to feeling freezing. On this occasion, the "physiological" framework exceeds the "mental" framework.

This asymmetry of causal impacts in mind systems has been underestimated. In any case, could systems that target intrinsic physiological instruments actuate top-down mental control? Developing research recommends that methods that consolidate physiologic stressors with focused reflection may "break" this asymmetry, permitting the mind to regulate the physiological. That is what we saw in late examinations we performed on the "Iceman" Wim Hof.

Hof's self-adjustment systems incorporate controlled breathing (hyperventilation and breath maintenance) and reflection. In our examination, he played out these systems before we more than once presented him to cold by siphoning super cold 39 °F water through an entire body wetsuit he wore.

Breath maintenance and cold structure are two physiologic stressors, though contemplation is a type of mental control. When typical subjects are presented to cold, internal heat level changes, activating homeostatic drives. Be that as it may, Hof's skin temperature stayed unaltered, unaffected by cool introduction. Besides, not at all like control subjects, he vigorously initiated the periaqueductal dim district of his mind, a territory significant for controlling agony. His self-educated strategy seems to change his cerebrum's capacity to manage cold by regulating torment pathways.

10 Things You Can Do to Change Your Brain Literally

We used to imagine that insight is inborn. A few people have it, and others simply don't. The cerebrum we're brought into the world with is the one we're left with forever.

That couldn't possibly be more off-base.

New and improving neuroscience advancements are giving us more profound knowledge into the secretive dark stuff between our ears. It turns out, our minds are shockingly unique; we accomplish things every day that influence their structure and science.

The following are ten of the manners in which we can change our cerebrums, regardless:

1. Working out

Physical action is significant for clear reasons. In any case, practice doesn't simply advance a more beneficial body. Ongoing research has demonstrated that physical exercise likewise benefits your cerebrum.

First off, physical activity can improve your cerebrum's "pliancy", a cerebral quality that influences memory, engine aptitudes, and the capacity to learn, as per a study led at the University of Adelaide in Australia. A little gathering of grown-ups in their late 20s and mid-30s took an interest in a 30-minute session of lively movement. Following the session, their cerebrums indicated a critical increment in neuroplasticity.

So, practice makes you more intelligent and more joyful simultaneously. Sounds like a successful win to me.

2. Resting

Rest is a fundamental movement that not even science can completely clarify. We realize that it's therapeutic, everybody does it, and an absence of it tends to be downright awful. In any case, specialists still battle to comprehend why we rest.

It surely isn't a vitality-sparing strategy, as we just really spare generally 50kCal through the span of an eight-hour rest. However, abandoning rest can make you crabby, lead to memory misfortune and bogus recollections, and, in extraordinary cases, cause slurred discourse and even cerebrum harm.

3. Ruminating

Individuals have depended on contemplation for centuries, and all things considered. Contemplation doesn't simply assist you with finding enthusiastic equalization in your life, it changes your cerebrum.

So, sitting still and attempting to concentrate on the present minute for as meager as 15 minutes out of each day fundamentally diminishes pressure and generally makes you a superior individual.

4. Drinking espresso

For quite a long-time, people have taken an interest in customizing taking seeds, simmering them, crushing them, and soaking the grounds in high temp water for a brisk shock of vitality. A few people won't get up without the guarantee of a warm cup of joe hanging tight for them. Be that as it may, what is this stimulating beverage truly doing to your cerebrum?

To summarize it, espresso (truly, caffeine) truly changes your cerebrum science, giving you that increase in vitality and center you need in the first part of the day. Be that as it may, likewise with anything, it's best with some restraint. (However, it is fairly ameliorating to realize it would take many cups of espresso in a brief timeframe to kill you.)

5. Perusing

Ever feel yourself escaping in a story, envisioning yourself in the shoes of the hero, and imagining the imaginary world around you? Losing all sense of direction in a book may lastingly affect your mind, says an examination of a study from Emory University.

6. Tuning in to music

When a few people need to center, they look for absolute quietness, however many turn on their music. Turns out, there's a logical explanation for this. Ben Greenfield clarifies:

When you diagram the electrical movement of your mind utilizing EEG, you create what is known as a brainwave design, which is known as a "wave" design in light of its cyclic, wave-like nature… When we bring down the cerebrum wave recurrence, we can place ourselves in a perfect condition to adapt new data, perform progressively expand assignments, learn dialects, and investigate complex circumstances. We can even be in what sports therapists call "The Zone", which is a condition of improved concentration and execution in athletic rivalries or exercise. Some portion of this is because being the somewhat diminished electrical movement in the cerebrum can prompt critical increments in feel-great mind synthetic substances like endorphins, norepinephrine, and dopamine.

Above all, you can really "power" your cerebrum into this perfect "alpha mind wave unwinding" with the correct recurrence of music.

7. Meandering in nature

Investing energy in open-air green spaces has been connected to enhancements in mindset, focus, and imagination. Presently an ongoing report has given us some knowledge into the neurological procedures that may be making these advantages.

8. Performing various tasks

A developing assortment of research has unmistakably demonstrated that people are physically unequipped for performing multiple tasks. Rather, the human cerebrum just takes single undertakings rapidly, exchanging to and from between various errands at a rate that makes you feel and accept you're completing two things on the double.

However, you aren't. Sorry to learn the unwanted messenger.

If you think you invest quite a bit of your energy "performing various tasks", you could be revamping your cerebrum, and not positively.

9. Eating sugar

Substantial sugar consumption made the rodents build up protection from insulin, a hormone that controls glucose levels and directs synapses' capacity. Insulin reinforces the synaptic associations between synapses, helping them convey better and structure more grounded recollections. So, when insulin levels in the cerebrum are brought down as the aftereffect of overabundance sugar utilization, cognizance can be weakened.

Along these lines, eating a lot of sugar can disable memory and learning abilities, and may add to neurodegenerative infections like Alzheimer's and dementia.

In any case, that is not all. Counting many of the sweet stuff in your eating routine has appeared to associate with the expanded danger of sorrow. Sugar initiates the state of mind improving synapse serotonin in our cerebrum. When ceaselessly overstimulated, our serotonin levels start to drain, making it progressively hard for us to manage our state of mind.

10. Trusting you can change your mind

At long last, for reasons unknown, basically accepting that you can change your cerebrum physically can in certainty assist you with changing your mind.

CHAPTER 2: YOUR BODY AND INTERMITTENT FASTING: ALL THE BENEFITS

Weight Loss

Intermittent fasting switches from periods of eating and to periods of fasting. Naturally, if you fast, your calorie intake will reduce, and it also helps you maintain your weight loss. It also prevents you from indulging in mindless eating. Whenever you eat something, your body converts the food into glucose and fat. It uses this glucose immediately and stores the fat for later use. When you skip a few meals, your body starts to reach into its internal stores of fat to provide energy. Also, most of the fat that you lose is from the abdominal region. If you want a flat tummy, then this is the perfect diet for you.

Tackles Diabetes

Diabetes is a significant threat on its own. It is also a primary indicator of the increase in risk factors of various cardiovascular diseases like heart attacks and strokes. When the glucose level increases alarmingly in the bloodstream, and there isn't enough insulin to process this glucose, it causes diabetes. When your body resists insulin, it becomes difficult to regulate insulin levels in the body. Intermittent fasting reduces insulin sensitivity and helps tackle diabetes.

Sleep

Lack of sleep is one of the main causes of obesity. When your body doesn't get enough sleep, the internal mechanism of burning fat suffers. Intermittent fasting regulates your sleep cycle and, in turn, makes your body effectively burn fats. A good sleep cycle has different physiological benefits; it makes you feel energetic and elevates your overall mood.

Resistance to Illnesses

Intermittent Fasting helps in the growth and regeneration of cells. Did you know that the human body has an internal mechanism that helps repair damaged cells? Intermittent fasting helps kickstart this mechanism. It improves the overall functioning of all the cells in the body. So, it is directly responsible for improving your body's natural defense mechanism by increasing its resistance to diseases and illnesses.

A Healthy Heart

Intermittent fasting assists in weight loss, and weight loss improves your cardiovascular health. A buildup of plaque in blood vessels is known as atherosclerosis. This is the primary cause of various cardiovascular diseases. The endothelium is the thin lining of blood vessels, and any dysfunction in it results in atherosclerosis. Obesity is the primary problem that plagues humanity and is also the main reason for the increase of plaque deposits in the blood vessels. Stress and inflammation also increase the severity of this problem. Intermittent fasting tackles the buildup of fat and helps tackle obesity. So, all you need to do is follow the simple protocols of Intermittent Fasting to improve your overall health.

A Healthy Gut

There are several millions of microorganisms present in your digestive system. These microorganisms help improve the overall functioning of your digestive system and are known as the gut microbiome. Intermittent Fasting enhances the health of these microbiomes and improves your digestive health. A healthy digestive system helps in better absorption of food and improves the functioning of your stomach.

Reduces Inflammation

Whenever your body feels there is an internal problem, its natural defense is inflammation. It doesn't mean that all forms of inflammation are desirable. Inflammation can cause several serious health conditions like arthritis, atherosclerosis, and other neurodegenerative disorders.

Any inflammation of this nature is known as chronic inflammation and is quite painful. Chronic inflammation can restrict your body's movements too. If you want to keep inflammation in check, then Intermittent Fasting will certainly come in handy.

Promotes Cell Repair

When you fast, the cells in your body start the process of waste removal. Waste removal means the breaking down of all dysfunctional cells and proteins and is known as autophagy. Autophagy offers protection against several degenerative diseases like Alzheimer's and cancer. You don't like accumulating garbage in your home, do you? Similarly, your body must not hold onto any unnecessary toxins. Autophagy is the body's way of getting rid of all things useless.

Higher Concentration and Brain Power

When subjected to food scarcity for a long time, mammals, including humans, will start to experience a decrease in their organ size. One of these organs is the brain. While some organs return to their original size over time, others may be impacted over the long term.

The brain handles the basic cognitive function of the body. To function properly and get the needed nutrients, it needs to return to its original size. However, if the brain becomes too foggy, getting the needed food nutrients will be pretty difficult, leading to malnutrition and even being fatal. However, during a shorter food scarcity period, the brain becomes hyperactive in its search for food as a mechanism for survival.

Excessive availability of food and eating altogether makes us mentally dull. Reflect on a time when you were completely satisfied after a big meal. After eating a massive plate of food, you will likely go into a "food coma" and curl up and sleep, or maybe just watch your favorite TV show on Netflix rather than get the motivation to go achieve your goals. Without a doubt, food satisfaction makes man naturally lose the drive to pursue his goals, which ultimately leads to dulling the brain. With this in mind, know that when you fast, your cognitive abilities are quickened. This improves your mental keenness, allowing you to achieve your health-related goals as opposed to excessively feeding.

It should be established here that there is no scientific research to support the notion that intermittent fasting alters mental alertness negatively. Fasting will not affect your cognitive function, such as moods, mental alertness, reaction time, intention, and sleep in any bad way. On the contrary, these things get boosted during fasting.

Fasting Promotes Autophagy and Protects Neurons

This is one of the many wondrous benefits of intermittent fasting, which many people should look forward to. Fasting is amazing in that it keeps the brain's cells from degeneration. This is because fasting prevents neural death.

Besides, fasting also triggers the process of autophagy in the brain, autophagy is the process in which the body gets rid of damaged body cells and brings out new ones. When the body is full of healthy, active, and improved cells, it is strong and well-equipped to combat any diseases that might want to attack.

With autophagy, the risk of viral infection and duplication of intracellular parasites reduces drastically. This dramatically reduces intracellular pathogens, such as cancer cells. Besides, the brain and other body tissue cells are protected from abnormal growth, inflammation, and toxicity.

Reduced Risk of Depression

With intermittent fasting, there is an increase in the levels of a neurotransmitter called a neurotrophic factor. When the body is deficient in this brain-derived factor, it contributes to significant depression and other mood disorders. Hence, intermittent fasting helps improve mental alertness and enhance mood, which ultimately leads to a reduced tendency to develop these conditions.

There are a couple of metabolic features that get triggered when we fast that improve brain health. This explains why people who practice intermittent fasting have lower inflammation levels, low blood sugar levels, and reduced oxidative stress.

There are also indications that intermittent fasting can keep the brain protected against the risk of stroke.

Intermittent Fasting Fosters Immune Regulation

When you fast, part of the body's primary aim is to keep the immune system healthy. This is why we encourage drinking a large quantity of water during the period of the intermittent fast, and afterward as well. Water can be spiced up with other detox agents that remove toxins from the digestive system and reduce unhealthy gut microbes. Keep in mind that the number of gut microbes present in the gastrointestinal tract is directly related to the immune system's function.

Intermittent fasting determines the number of inflammatory cytokines that the body has. Hence, it helps regulate the body's overall immune system. In the body, we have two significant cytokines that cause inflammation in the body: Interleukin-6 and Tumor Necrosis Factor Alpha. Fasting suppresses the release of these inflammatory pro-inflammatory cytokines.

Intermittent Fasting Reduces the Risk of Chronic Disease

People living with chronic autoimmune diseases like Crohn's disease, colitis, rheumatoid arthritis, and systemic lupus will definitely see remarkable improvement with intermittent fasting. The idea is simple. Fasting reduces the rate of an extreme inflammatory process in the bodies of these persons. With this, they have an ideal immune function.

For instance, cancer cells have between ten and seventy extra insulin receptors in contrast to healthy body cells. This happens as a result of the breakdown of sugar for fuel. With intermittent fasting, cancer cells are starved of sugar intake. This conditions the cells for damage through free radicals.

Improves Genetic Repair Mechanisms

The tendency of the body to live longer increases when it does not get enough food. This is because, with intermittent fasting, there is repair and regeneration of cells that come about via a repair mechanism in the body. This is understandable, as the energy required for cell repair is lesser when compared to what is necessary for cell creation or division.

Hence, during the period of intermittent fasting, cell division, and creation in the body becomes reduced. This is a necessary process, vital especially for the healing of malignant cells, which thrive as a result of abnormal cell division.

In the body, the human growth hormone (HGH) takes care of the process of cell repair. It is a human growth hormone that brings about changes in metabolism that cause tissue repair and fat burning. Thus, when we fast, the body can concentrate more on repairing body tissues with amino acids and enzymes. This restores tissue collagen and also triggers an improvement in bones, ligaments, tendons, and general muscle function in the body.

Reduce the Likelihood of Developing Cancer

Lastly, studies have found that intermittent can reduce your likelihood of developing cancer and help make treatment more successful. As you are aware, intermittent fasting can help treat oxidative stress and cellular damage, both of which cause cancer. By reducing this damage, you can thereby reduce your risk of developing cancer in the future.

But that is not all. While human studies still need to be conducted, a study on mice found that when practicing short-term fasting chemotherapy treatment becomes more successful in targeting and treating both breast cancer and skin cancer. Not only did the chemotherapy itself become more effective, but the mice' immune systems also were better able to fight off the cancerous cells and growths, which is essential as chemotherapy is well-known for reducing a person's immune system drastically.

CHAPTER 3: KINDS OF INTERMITTENT FASTING: 16/8, 20/4, 23/1, AND MORE

16/8 Method

This's just about the most popular fasting methods since it's so schedule-based, meaning there are no surprises. This will give you the freedom to control when you eat based on the everyday life of yours. The 16 is the number of hours you're likely to be fasting, which may also be lowered to 12 or perhaps 14 hours if that fits into your life better. Then you're eating period is going to be between 8 and 10 hours every day. This might seem daunting, but it just means that you are skipping an entire meal. Many people choose to begin their fast around 7 or 8 p.m. and then do not eat until 11 or noon the next day, which means they fast for the recommended 16 hours. Of course, it isn't as bad as it sounds since they are sleeping during this time, so what it comes down to is eating dinner and then not eating again the next day around lunch, so you are just skipping breakfast.

You will be doing it every day, so finding the hours that work for you are important. If you work the third shift, then switching you're eating period around to fit into your schedule is important. If you find yourself being run down and sluggish, tweak your fasting hours until you find a healthy balance. Granted, there will be some adjustment, because, chances are, your body is not accustomed to skipping entire meals. However, this should go away after a couple of weeks, and if it doesn't, then try starting your fasting period earlier in the day, allowing you to eat earlier the next or alter it however you need to feel healthy and happy.

Lean-Gains Method (14:10)

The lean-gains method has several different incarnations on the web, but its fame comes from the fact that it helps shed fat while building it into muscle almost immediately. Through the lean-gains method, you'll find yourself able to shift all that fat to be muscle through a rigorous practice of fasting, eating right, and exercising.

Through this method, you fast anywhere from 14 to 16 hours and spend the remaining 10 or 8 hours each day engaged in eating and exercise. As opposed to the crescendo, this method features daily fasting and eating, rather than alternated days of eating versus not. Therefore, you don't have to be quite cautious about extending the physical effort to exercise on the days you are fasting because those days when you're fasting are every day!

For the lean-gaining method, start fasting only for 14 hours and work it up to 16 if you feel comfortable with it, but never forget to drink enough water and be careful about spending too much energy on exercise! Remember that you want to grow in health and potential through intermittent fasting. You'll certainly not want to lose any of that growth by forcing the process along.

20:4 Method

Stepping things up a notch from the 14:10, and 16:8 methods, the 20:4 method is a tough one to master, for it is rather unforgiving. People talk about this method of intermittent fasting as intense and highly restrictive. Still, they also say that the effects of living this method are almost unparalleled with all other tactics.

For the 20:4 method, you'll fast for 20 hours each day and squeeze all your meals, all your eating, and all your snacking into 4 hours. People who attempt 20:4 normally have two smaller meals or just one large meal, and a few snacks during their 4-hour window to eat, and it is up to the individual which four hours of the day they devote to eating.

The trick for this method is to make sure you're not overeating or bingeing during those 4-hour windows to eat. It is all-too-easy to get hungry during the 20-hour fast, and have that feeling then propel you into intense and unrealistic hunger or meal sizes after the fast period is over. Be careful if you try this method. If you're new to intermittent fasting, work your way up to this one gradually, and if you're working your way up already, only make the shift to 20:4 when you know you're ready. It would surely disappoint if all your progress with intermittent fasting got hijacked by one poorly thought-out goal with the 20:4 method.

Meal Skipping

Meal skipping is an extremely flexible form of intermittent fasting that can provide all of the benefits of intermittent fasting, but with less strict scheduling. If you are not someone who has a typical schedule or feels like a stricter variation of the intermittent fasting diet will serve you, meal skipping is a viable alternative.

Many people who choose to use meal skipping find it a great way to listen to their bodies and follow their basic instincts. If they are not hungry, they simply don't eat that meal. Instead, they wait for the next one. Meal skipping can also help people who have time constraints, and who may not always be able to get in a certain meal of the day.

It is important to realize that with meal skipping, you may not always be maintaining a 10-16-hour window of fasting. As a result, you may not get every benefit that comes from other fasting diets. However, this may be a great solution for people who want an intermittent fasting diet that feels more natural. It may also be a great idea for those looking to begin listening to their bodies more so that they can adjust to a more intense variation of the diet with greater ease. It can be a great transitional diet for you if you are not ready to jump into one of the other fasting diets just yet.

Eat-Stop-Eat (24 Hour) Method

This method of fasting is incredibly similar to the crescendo method. The only discernable difference is that there's no anticipation of increasing into a more intense fasting pattern with time. For the eat-stop-eat method, you decide which days you want to take off from eating, and then you run with it until you've lost that weight, and then you keep running with the lifestyle for good because you won't be able to imagine life without it.

The eat-stop-eat method involves one to two days a week being 100% oriented towards fasting, with the other five to six days concerning "business as normal." The one or two days spent fasting are then full 24-hour days spent without eating anything at all. These days, of course, water and coffee are still fine to drink, but no food items can be consumed whatsoever. Exercise is also frowned upon on those fasting days but see what your body can handle before you decide how that should all work out.

Some people might start thinking they're using the crescendo method, but end up sticking with eat-stop-eat.

Alternate-Day Method

The alternate-day method is admittedly a little confusing, but the reason it could be so confusing could come, in part, from how much wiggle room it provides for the practitioner. This method is great for people who don't have a consistent schedule or any sense of one; it is incredibly forgiving for those who don't quite have everything together for themselves yet.

When it comes down to it, alternate-day intermittent fasting is really up to you. You should try to fast every other day, but it doesn't have to be that precise. Similarly, with the crescendo method, as long as you fast two to three days a week, with a break day or two in between each fasting day, you're set! Then, you'll want to eat normally for three or four days out of each week, and when you encounter a fasting day, you don't even need to completely fast!

Alternate-day fasting is a solid place to start from, especially if you work a varying schedule or still have yet to get used to a consistent one. If you want to make things more intense from this starting point, the alternate-day method can easily become the eat-stop-eat method, the crescendo method, or the 5:2 method. Essentially, this method is a great place to begin

12:12 Method

As another of the more natural ways of intermittent fasting, the 12:12 approach is well-suited to beginning practitioners. Many people live out the 12:12 method without any forethought simply because of their sleeping and eating schedule, but turning 12:12 into a conscious practice can have just as many positive effects on your life as the more drastic 20:4 method claims.

According to a study conducted in the University of Alabama for this method, in particular, you fast for 12 hours and then enter a 12-hour eating window. It's not difficult whatsoever to get three small meals and several snacks, or two big meals and a snack into your day with this method. With 12:12, the standard meal timing works just fine.

Ultimately, this method is a great one to start from, for a lot of variation can be built into this scheduling when you're ready to make things more interesting. Effortlessly and without much effort, 12:12 can become 14:10 or even 16:8, and in seemingly no time, you can find yourself trying alternate-day or crescendo methods, too. Start with what's normal for you, and this method might be exactly that!

5:2 Method

This is another popular way to fast, because there is no true fasting involved, but instead a strict and drastic reduction of calories for two days each week. So, for five days a week, you will eat your normal 1.600 to 2,000 calories and exercise like normal. The on two nonconsecutive days a week, you will restrict your caloric intake to between 500 and 600 calories. When doing this, pay close attention to the number of calories in beverages as well, many people make the mistake of only counting calories in what they eat. Remember, that beverages contain calories too, especially if you are drinking things from coffee shops, as these tend to have high amounts of sugar.

Crescendo Method

This is usually an introduction to fasting; it is how many people begin their fasting journey. This is a less intense form of intermittent fasting and is a great way for you to see how it works to ease your fears and become familiarized with a fasting schedule. This method involves normally 4 or 5 days a week and then restricting you're eating period to between 8 or 10 hours for two or three nonconsecutive days. Very similar to the 16/8 method, but instead of doing it every day, you only do it a couple of days each week. These are the safest ways for women to fast because they do not upset the body's hormonal balance. Intermittent fasting not done properly can trick the body into going into what is known as starvation mode. This happens when the body thinks it needs to hold onto fat longer because it doesn't know when it will have a chance to consume food for fuel again. This can lead to burning muscle for fuel and upsetting the hormonal balance, leading to even more issues. However, intermittent fasting done properly can be safe and incredibly beneficial.

Intermittent fasting helps you lose weight, but it also improves mental clarity and simplifies your life in a way that diets do not. Consider the length of time spent worrying about or perhaps eating food, and then imagine what other things you can be doing if this weren't the case. This's one of the main benefits of intermittent fasting; you will find no surprises and can take total control of when you eat.

CHAPTER 4: INTERMITTENT FASTING AND SUPPLEMENTS

Not all supplements can provide the health benefits you need. Taking the wrong supplements, especially while you are on intermittent fasting, may bring harm. The right types of health supplements can significantly boost the effects of intermittent fasting.

We will briefly discuss the problems with taking generic supplements, how to choose the right health supplements for those who are into intermittent fasting, and a comprehensive list of health supplements that you should take.

The Problem with Multivitamins

Multivitamins are very popular. Millions of people around the world are taking multivitamins, so people think that they are indispensable for fighting disease and malnutrition. This is, in fact, a misconception. In reality, not everyone can benefit from multivitamins and instead choose targeted supplements.

Nutritional Imbalance

Many multivitamins contain too many specific nutrients, such as Vitamin A or C, and not enough of the other essential nutrients such as magnesium.

So, there is a tendency to overdose on a few nutrients and not taking enough of the others.

Some manufacturers still include a long list of multivitamins on their labels, but the truth is, some of these vitamins are in very small amounts. Many consumers ignore the insubstantial amounts of important nutrients. How can you fit a range of nutrients in only one pill? Also, we need to consider the nutritional needs of each person. A bodybuilder will require a different set of nutrients compared to a lactating mom.

Low Quality of Multivitamins

Each type of nutrient behaves differently inside the body. While folate is an important B vitamin, folic acid, the form found in generic multivitamins, may increase the risk of colon cancer according to a study published by the University of Chile.

This could be the reason why some researches, such as a 2009 study published by the University of East Finland, suggest a connection between multivitamins and an increase in mortality, while another research commissioned by the American Medical Association in 2009 reveals no benefit in taking multivitamins.

Furthermore, many multivitamins are manufactured with additives and fillers, which make it difficult for the body to absorb nutrients. Therefore, a minimal amount of important nutrients may reach your cells.

We are actually getting what we pay for with multivitamins. You may convince yourself and choose the generic multivitamins in the store, or you may add a bit and actually choose targeted supplements to help improve your health.

Supplements and Fasting

Eating whole and natural foods are still the best source to get the important nutrients that our body needs. Remember, whole foods may behave differently from their individual components. For example, the nutrients from a piece of broccoli are more accessible compared to consuming an equal amount of nutrients from a powder or a pill.

The antioxidants sourced from natural foods are beneficial, but consuming mega doses of some synthetic antioxidants may come with risks such as the growth of tumors based on a 1993 toxicology research from the University of Hamburg.

Food synergy enables the nutrients in food to work together. Hence, food is more powerful compared to its components. This is why it is crucial to begin with a diet that is rich in nutrients, then add supplements that are based on your goals and needs.

It is important to take note that just because something is natural doesn't mean it is helpful. There is a tendency for some, especially the health buffs, to abuse even food-based vitamins and herbal supplements.

These supplements are still vulnerable to contaminants and heavy metals from manufacturing. Be sure to check the sourcing and quality testing of your supplements. It is ideal to check with a licensed professional who can recommend safe brands of supplements.

CHAPTER 5: INTERMITTENT FASTING: STEP-BY-STEP

There are a few things you have to remember whether you need to shed pounds with intermittent fasting, here below the main four:

- *Food quality:* The food you eat is still important. Try to eat whole and simply seasoned foods.

- *Calories:* Calories, despite everything, still count. Try to eat "typically" during the eating periods and not to make up for the calories you missed by fasting.

- *Consistency:* Just like any other weight loss strategy, you have to stick with it for a long term if you want it to work.

- *Patience:* It will take as much time as is needed to get used to an intermittent fasting lifestyle. Try to be consistent with your meal calendar, and it will get simpler.

The greater part of the famous intermittent fasting methods also suggests food quality. This is significant in case you need to lose body fat while keeping muscle.

In the beginning, calorie counting is commonly not required with intermittent fasting. If your weight loss slows down, then, calorie counting can be a useful practice.

With intermittent fasting, you, despite everything, need to eat healthily and keep up a calorie shortage if you need to get in shape.

Defining Specific Measurable Goals

Rather than setting a general goal like "getting more fit", be more specific, focus on basic, feasible objectives that should be possible week by week, like:

- Taking a walk three days per week
- Drink 64 ounces of water per day, every day, this week
- Skip one meal this week

Self-Reward When Reaching Small Targets

Set yourself up for progress by utilizing a prize framework. For example:

- After shedding 15 pounds, get yourself some new clothes.
- If you meet all your monthly goals, treat yourself to a massage

The cash spared by skipping a meal (or two) can pay for your prize! Things that can motivate us are different for every one of us, so make sure to find out what might work best for you, and you will stay focused on reaching all of your goals.

Keeping a Journal

This is quite a game-changer. If you have very strong will power, and you are used to doing medium to long term plans and stick to them, you probably won't need to keep a journal, if not for the pleasure to do it, and unless this already is one of the tools behind your willpower.

Most of us though are not like this. The ability to stick to a plan (dietary or of any other nature) is seldom a talent. More often than you think, there are tools and practices involved. When it comes to diets, especially, but not only, if the aim is to lose weight, the number one cause of quitting is the lack of immediate and measurable results. Or at least, this is the reason the quitter, in all honesty, gives. But it really is about this? Well, not exactly. Most of the time, it is not that one does not have results, it is that they have in mind the big final goal, therefore they can't appreciate the small ones during the journey.

If your final goal is to save 10.000 dollars, you won't get excited about your first 10 dollars saved. If your final goal is to lift 200 pounds, you won't get excited about your first 20 pounds lifted. If your final goal is to shed 20 pounds, you won't get excited about your first 10 ounces shed. But the truth is, to save 10.000 dollars, to lift 200 pounds, to shed 20 pounds; you have to start saving 10, lifting 20, shedding just your first 10 ounces.

This is the main use of journaling: keeping track day by day of the small victories to celebrate and the small struggles to fight, being able to have everything under control and to love and appreciate the journey, until you won't need to keep track anymore and either will quit doing it or will keep on just for the pleasure of it.

Once you know what to keep track of, it is very easy, and pleasant, to do it. Not only it is the chance to track your progress, but it also is something that gives you a moment that is all yours, where you can in some way talk to yourself.

I usually suggest setting a "three months challenge" because this is, give or take, the period of time in which you may see yourself as a "beginner" of intermittent fasting. Usually, after three months you are in the zone, you just acquired the intermittent fasting lifestyle as your own, and you don't need to journal about it anymore (of course you can, someone does it, but it becomes more of a pleasure than a tool).

6 Ways to Make A Fast Diet Effective

1. Know your weight, BMI, and waist size from the start

As mentioned earlier, the waist measurement is an essential and straightforward measure of internal fat and a strong predictor of future health. People with intermittent fasting quickly lose those dangerous and unattractive centimeters. The BMI is the square of the weight (in kilograms) divided by the height (in meters). It looks ugly and may sound abstract, but it is a widely used tool to find a way to healthy weight loss. The BMI values do not take into account your body type, age, or ethnicity. You should, therefore, greet them informed. However, this is useful when you need a number.

Weigh yourself regularly. After the first phases, once a week is sufficient. If you want the numbers to drop, the morning after fasting is your best bet. Researchers at the University of Illinois noted: "Weighing can vary significantly from food to fasting days. This weight deviation is probably due to the extra weight of food in the digestive tract.

It is not a daily change in fat mass. Future solutions may require solutions that try averaging the weight measurements on consecutive feeding and fasting days to determine weight more accurately. There are 28 tasks. If you are a person who likes structure and clarity, you may want to track your progress. Think about your goals. When and where do you want to go? Be realistic: rapid weight loss is not recommended. Please take your time. Make a plan. Write it down.

Many people recommend keeping a diet journal. Add your experience next to the number. Note the three good things that happen every day. It is a message of happiness that can be referenced over time.

2.   Find a quick friend

You need very few accessories to be successful, but a supportive friend can be one of them. Once you are on the fast diet, tell people about it; you may find that they join you, and you will build a network of shared experiences. As the plan appeals to both men and women, couples report that doing it together is more comfortable. This way, you get mutual support, camaraderie, shared engagement, and shared anecdotes. Also, mealtimes are infinitely more comfortable if you eat with someone who understands the basics of the plot.

There are also many discussions in online discussion forums. A mum net is an excellent source of support and information. It is remarkable how reassuring it is to know that you are not alone.

3. Quick meal preparation

Prepare your quick meal in advance, so you do not have to search for food and come across a sausage that irresistibly hides in the fridge. Keep it simple and effortlessly strive for the taste of the day. Buy and cook on non-fast days to avoid laughing at inappropriate temptations. Clean the house of junk food before embarking. It will only sing and coo in the closets, making your fasting day more difficult than it should be.

4. Check the partial size of the calorie label

If the serial box says "30 g", weigh it. Continue. Be surprised. Then be honest. Your calorie count is necessarily fixed and limited on an empty stomach, so it is important not to worry about how much is flowing. Here, you'll find our recommended fast food calorie counters. More importantly, do not count calories on late days.

You have better things. Wait before you eat. Resist at least 10 minutes, and preferably 15 minutes, to see if your hunger subsides (which is usually the case). If you need a snack, choose one that does not raise your insulin levels. Try carrot carrots, a handful of popcorn, apple slices, or strawberries. But do not pinch like chicken all day. Calories are stacked up quickly, and your fasting is fast. Eat consciously on a fasting day and fully absorb the fact that you are eating (especially if you have ever been in a massive traffic jam). Also, be careful with your vacation. Do not eat until you are satisfied (of course, this happens after a few weeks of practice).

Find out what the concept of "satisfaction" means to you. We are all different, and it changes over time.

5. Stay busy

"We humans are always looking for activities between meals," Leonard Cohen said. Yes, see where it takes us. So, fill your day, not your face. "No one is hungry during the first few seconds of skydiving," said Brad Pilon, the advocate of fasting. Distraction is the best defense against the dark art of the food industry, with doughnuts and nachos on every corner. If you need this doughnut, keep in mind that it will remain tomorrow.

6. Try 2 to 2

Fast from 2:00 p.m. to 2:00 p.m., not from bedtime to bedtime. After lunch on the first day, eat modestly until late lunch on the next day.

This way, you will lose weight during sleep and will not feel uncomfortable for a day without food. This is a smart trick, but it requires a bit more focus than the all-day option. Alternatively, you can go from dinner to dinner quickly. In short, no day is fast and fun. The point is that this plan is "adapted to adjustment." Just like your waist.

Get Started

1. Determine the start date

We strongly recommend starting on Monday. It makes more sense. After you have selected a day, you can thoroughly prepare for the start time with a few steps.

2. Select the distribution of fast / meal to determine when to eat and fast

16/8 is recommended for beginners. You have to get used to it a lot, and it is not too difficult the first time. Select a window and decide when to stop eating the night before fasting. It will serve as a separate house. We recommend that you stick to it for the first week. After practicing FI for a few weeks, it is only natural to change windows and schedules. However, it is best to keep the same time during the first week. So, if you stop eating at 9 p.m. on Sunday, you won't eat at 1 p.m. on Monday. From 1 p.m. to 9 p.m., it will be a dining room window.

3. Spend a flirt day

Spend one day on the day before the first fast. Eat a lot and eat whatever you like. It has two purposes. First, the more foods there are in the system, the easier it is to make fast-first. Secondly, if you eat the things you want the night before, that means you won't thirst for these foods for a week.

4. Teach people

I highly recommend talking to your loved ones about the new habits you are adopting. Explain why you do it, and why you are hired-politely informed them that you do not eat at certain times and that you will like their support, please. Warn people to make up for your chances of getting food during a fast. One of the most difficult challenges you face is that of a friend, family, or colleague who provides you with food-inform your FI and avoids it.

5. Buy branched-chain amino acids (optional)

Branched-chain amino acids (BCAA) are beneficial on an empty stomach. These are pure forms of protein and incredibly powerful for more prolonged fasting. Consuming 10 g of BCAAs can help reduce hunger without fasting. Do not exceed 10 g per serving, but two servings are sufficient during fasting. If you want to exercise, I recommend BCAA. If you are going to exercise, we recommend that you exercise 60 minutes before and during exercise at one of the following times.

6. Training and intermittent fasting

You do not have to exercise to take advantage of intermittent fasting. However, when you select training, you'll see unprecedented levels of results. As explained earlier in this book, it increases growth hormone and testosterone production and attacks adipocytes, and stores. With the addition of an exercise routine (we recommend strength training), the results you see are incredible. Strength training combined with increased hormones can help you build muscle faster than expected. Lifting weights also increases the production of testosterone and growth hormone, so your body receives twice the dose of hormone production. Weight training is also very metabolic, so shred fat from your body and remember, as I said, you have more muscles, which means less fat.

I would also like to mention that strength training and exercise are probably the most effective way to protect your body from whatever the world throws at you. It has been proven to reduce stress, help with depression, increase energy levels, improve mental function, increase your happiness, improve your life, and help you live longer. Therefore, it is highly recommended to start training. If you do not have a good gym, strength exercises like pushups, squats, and lunges can help you on your journey. Finally, I would like to add one thing, if it can be speeded up, run it. I understand that planning does not mean everyone can do it, but one way to improve is to exercise and fast with a meal after exercise. Do not eat more than 2 hours after weight training, as your muscles will be disrupted, and this will negatively affect your goals.

CHAPTER 6: WHAT TO DRINK DURING FASTING?

Beverages for Hydration in Intermittent Fasting

- Sparkling water
- Watermelon
- Strawberries
- Oranges
- Water
- Cantaloupe
- Peaches
- Lettuce
- Celery
- Black coffee or tea
- Tomatoes
- Cucumber
- Skim milk
- Plain yogurt

Water

Essentially, water is not food, but it's an essential one to get through it. Basically, for any significant organ in the body, water is vital to wellbeing. As part of the fast, you will be reckless to stop drinking water. The organs are pretty significant. Depending on gender, height, activity level, weight, and environment, the amount of water each person can drink differs. But a reasonable indicator is your urine color. For all times, you like it to be pale yellow.

Dehydration indicates dark yellow urine, which may induce headaches, exhaustion, and lightheadedness. Couple it with minimal food, and you've got a catastrophe formula, or rather dark pee, for the very least. Add a splash of lemon juice, a few mint leaves, or any cucumber slices to the water if the prospect of pure water does not excite you. Promoting hydration is among the most critical ways of sustaining a balanced eating routine when fasting intermittently.

When you go for 12-16 hours without food, the sugar contained in the liver, also known as glycogen, is the main source of energy for the body. When this energy is burned, a huge number of electrolytes and fluid dissolve. During the intermittent fasting regimen, consuming at least 8 cups of water a day can reduce dehydration and encourage improved cognition, blood flow, and joint muscle and support.

Coffee

What about a nice cup of hot coffee? Do not worry; Coffee is allowed. Since coffee is a calorie-free product in its natural form, it may also be drunk beyond a specified feeding window. But if you add creamers, syrups, or any flavorings, it cannot be drunk at the duration of the fast. Keep that in mind and enjoy coffee

Fresh Smoothies

Try jumping to a double dose of vitamins by making organic smoothies filled with fresh vegetables and fruits if a daily supplement doesn't suit you. Smoothies are a perfect way to ingest diverse foods, each filled with various essential nutrients especially. Buy frozen fruits to save money and for ultimate delicious recipes.

Fortified Milk with Vitamin D

The average calcium consumption is 1,000 mg a day for an adult, exactly what you can receive from consuming three cups of milk a day. The opportunities to drink this much may be scarce with a shortened feeding window, so it is necessary to choose high-calcium foods. Vitamin D fortified milk increases calcium absorption by the body. It helps maintain bones healthy. One should add milk to cereal or smoothies or even just consume it with foods to improve the regular calcium intake. Non-dairy options rich in calcium contain tofu and soy goods, as well as leafy greens, including kale.

CHAPTER 7: WHAT TO EAT AFTER FASTING?

Food always plays a very important role in our overall health. The health debacle that we are facing these days has two important parts:

- Our Eating Habits
- The Things We Eat

Our Eating Habits

This is a very important part because poor eating habits and reckless eating can damage our whole food processing and energy management system. Intermittent fasting is the answer to poor eating habits as it can help you in improving your food intake.

This is helpful to a great extent. Intermittent fasting relies on managing your eating habits to such a great extent that if you can manage your eating habits properly, you can eat anything you like in moderation.

This can seem to be a great exaggeration for the people who have been following punishing diets all their lives. Cycles of restrictions, endless temptations, and events of binge eating are the major phases in their lives.

Intermittent fasting doesn't pose such restrictions. If you are feeling compelled to eat the cake your friend is offering you, you may go ahead and have a bite of it in your eating window without developing any guilt.

This is not to say that cake is not unhealthy. It is made up of refined carbs, refined sugar, and unhealthy fats. However, as long as you are eating it in moderation, you will be able to avoid major issues in your weight loss journey.

A big reason woman on punishing diets is not able to lose weight is their endless temptation for the forbidden things. It is very human to desire the things that you can't have, especially food. Diets put too many restrictions, and hence the dieters always feel tempted, and that poses emotional, physical, and psychological challenges. They can't eat anything they like without feeling the guilt inside them.

Intermittent fasting frees you from any such guilt. It allows you to eat the things you like in moderation so that there is no long-term temptation that may lead to binge eating or psychological barriers in the end.

The Things We Eat

The things we eat do play a role in our health. You can offset the harmful effects of some food products by not consuming them in large quantities, but that doesn't make them good or healthy.

- There are a few things that you should eat in good quantities.
- There are a few things that you may only eat in moderation.
- There are a few things that you must avoid.

Macronutrients

Fat, proteins, and carbohydrates are the three macronutrients, and you must have them in balanced quantities. Trapped in our fast-paced lives, we seldom pay attention to the macronutrients in food and their importance in our health. If you do not consume the three macronutrients in healthy proportions, you may find it very difficult to control your hunger, cravings, and energy levels. Imbalanced intake of these macronutrients can also lead to faster satiety and faster hunger pangs. You may also feel energy drained.

If you want to follow a healthy intermittent fasting routine, you must have a balanced meal in the following proportions.

Fat: 50-70%

The fat must constitute the highest part of your diet if you want to lose weight faster and have a better fasting routine. This may sound counterproductive as you are trying to lose fat, but there is no relation between eating healthy fat and gaining fat. As long as you are consuming healthy fats within your calorie limits, you will be losing weight just fine. Not only this, but healthy fats are also beneficial in lowering the risk of heart disorders and chronic inflammations.

- **Nuts and Seeds**: Almonds, walnuts, flax seeds, and chia seeds, are great sources of healthy fats.
- **Fatty fish:** Wild-caught fatty fish provide a lot of healthy fat. They are also a rich source of Omega3 fatty acids.

- **Eggs:** Egg is among the finest sources of fats. The egg yolk provides very healthy fat and can be consumed safely.

- **Avocado:** It is also a very good source of healthy fat.

- **Olive oil:** It is a good option to be used for cooking. However, even using too much olive oil can be harmful. You must use it in moderation.

Fat in your diet should be the highest if you want your body to get into ketosis. If you keep consuming too many carbs, even though your calorie intake may remain low, you'd always face difficulty in burning fat.

Another difficulty in consuming too many carbs is that they burn faster, and you may start having cravings too fast, and remaining in the fasting state may become difficult. The fat is a slow-burning fuel, and hence it takes much longer to get processed, therefore you wouldn't feel hunger pangs fast.

Protein: 15-25%

Protein in the diet is very important as our body can't produce protein. You will have to consume protein to compensate for all the loss of tissues, muscles, and the structural repair work in the body. Therefore, it is a macronutrient that isn't optional. However, although protein is so important, you can't have a lot of it.

If you are not doing serious physical work that involves a lot of muscle or tissue damage, your protein requirements would be moderate. Any excess protein consumed would be converted to carbs, and hence there would be an imbalance in your diet.

You can get healthy proteins from:

- Lean meats
- Legumes
- Pulses
- Egg whites
- White meat poultry
- Lean cuts of meat
- Soy
- Seafood

Striking a healthy balance with protein is very important. It can be crucial to your fasting routine as well. Protein takes the longest to get processed in the gut, and hence it keeps your digestive system engaged. If you are consuming protein in a balanced manner, you are less likely to feel hungry very often.

Carbohydrate 5-10%

Carbs are a major part of the modern diet. Our diet is filled with refined flours, refined sugar, processed food items, etc. They have a lot of carbs. Not only this, but most of our staple food items are also carb-rich, and hence we feel trapped when we are asked to lower our carb intake.

However, this is a mental limitation we have created. There are a lot of carbs that are healthy and can be consumed without any limitation.

Within carbs, there is a distinction between good carbs and bad carbs, and you must make that distinction in mind.

Bad Carbs

- **All Refined Flours:** You must not consume food items made up of refined flours. You must make it a habit to read the food labels carefully.

- **Refined Sugar:** Things made up of refined sugar must be eliminated from the diet. They will lead to food cravings and cause serious health issues.

- **Empty Calories:** This is the third category you must stay away from. All the processed items that are made up of maple syrup, fructose, or sugar must be avoided at all costs. You must also avoid carbonated beverages, sweetened beverages, fruit juices, and even fresh fruit juices. Most people have a misconception in their minds that fresh fruit juices are nutritious, but they are wrong. They only have calories and some vitamins, but they are devoid of all the minerals that your body needed. You must also avoid alcohol or other such things that have lots of concentrated carbs.

These things lead to a glucose spike in your bloodstream, invoking an immediate and heavy insulin response, but they do not offer anything to your gut. Your gut starts releasing gastric juices in anticipation but gets nothing in return. As a result, you may develop acid reflux, ulcer, and other such issues. The glucose spike in your bloodstream is also temporary as your body lowers the glucose level rapidly, and you soon start feeling the urge to have something to eat.

This is a reason you feel very good when you eat sugar-rich foods but start feeling energy devoid very soon.

Good Carbs

- ***Whole Grains:*** Whole grains are undoubtedly great for your gut as well as your body, and you must have them in smaller quantities. Whole grains have a lot of trace minerals that are important for your body, and you can't get them from other sources. Apart from that, they are a rich source of indigestible fiber that is very helpful in scrubbing your intestines clean.

- ***Non-starchy Leafy Greens:*** You can have non-starchy leafy greens as much as you want without thinking about your calorie intake. They are full of vitamins and antioxidants. Leafy greens are filling, and hence they will keep your stomach occupied without providing too many calories, and you wouldn't even feel hungry very often. Apart from that, leafy greens are full of soluble fiber that gets converted into a gel-like substance in your gut and cleanses your digestive system softly. It is very helpful and hence must be consumed in good quantities.

- ***Salads and Fruits:*** You can have salads and fruits in healthy quantities as they are also a rich source of fiber. You must try to have as much fiber as possible because it keeps your digestive system engaged, clean, and healthy.

CHAPTER 8: PHYSICAL EXERCISE AND FASTING

Many people will ask if it is safe to combine fasting with exercise. I am here to say it is. However, some factors need to be considered before combining the two. First, the type of fasting regimen should be considered alongside the physical, mental, and psychological health of the individual. Women with existing medical conditions should not combine fasting with exercises before being advised by a medical expert. So, while it is safe to practice intermittent fasting and include exercise if you are an already active person, doing so is not suitable for everyone.

First of all, your metabolism can be negatively impacted if you exercise and fast for long periods. For example, if you exercise daily while fasting for more than a month, your metabolic rate can begin to slow down. So, while it may sound like a quick way to reap the benefits of your limited calorie intake, moderation is crucial.

Combining the two can trigger a higher rate of breaking down glycogen and body fat. This means that you burn fat at an accelerated rate. Also, when you combine these two, your growth hormones are boosted. This results in improved bone density. Your muscles are also positively impacted when you exercise. Your muscles will become more resilient to stress and age slower. This is also a quick way to trigger autophagy keeping brain cells and tissues strong, making you feel and look younger.

Exercise is Even Better After 50

Cardiovascular exercise is great for the heart and lungs. It improves oxygen delivery to specific parts of your body, reduces stress, improves sleep, burns fat, and improves sex drive. Some of the more common cardio exercises are running, brisk walking, and swimming. In the gym, machines such as the elliptical, treadmill, and Stairmaster are used to help with cardio. Some people are satisfied and feel like they've done enough after 20 minutes on the treadmill, but if you want to continue to be strong and independent as you grow older; you need to consider adding strength training to your workout. After 50, strength training for a woman is no longer about six-pack abs, building biceps, or vanity muscles. Instead, it has switched to maintaining a body that is healthy, strong, and is less prone to injury and illness.

Women over 50 who engage in strength training for 20 to 30 minutes a day can reap the following benefits:

- **Reduced body fat:** Accumulating excess body fat is not healthy for any woman at any age. To prevent many of the diseases associated with aging, it is important to maintain a healthy body weight by burning excess fat.

- **Build bone density:** With stronger bones, accidental falls are less likely to result in broken limbs or a visit to the emergency room.

- **Build muscle mass:** Although you are not likely to be the next champion bodybuilder, strength training will make you an overall stronger woman who will carry herself with ease, push your lawnmower, lift your groceries, and perform all other tasks that require you to exert some strength.

- ***Significant less risk of chronic diseases:*** In addition to keeping chronic diseases away, strength training can also reduce symptoms of some diseases you may have, such as back pain, obesity, arthritis, osteoporosis, and diabetes. Of course, the type of exercises you do if you have any chronic disease should be recommended by your doctor.

- ***Boosts mental health:*** A loss of self-confidence and depression are some psychological issues that come along with aging. Women who keep themselves fit with exercises tend to be generally more self-assured and are less likely to develop depression.

Strength Training Exercises for Women Over 50

These ten-strength training exercises you can do right in the comfort of your home. All you need is a mat, a chair, and some hand weights of about 3 – 8 pounds. As you get stronger, you can increase the weight. Take a minute to rest before switching between each routine. Ensure that you move slowly through the exercises, breathe properly, and focus on maintaining the right form. If you start to feel lightheaded or dizzy during your routines, especially if you are performing the exercise during your fasting window, discontinue immediately.

Squat to Chair

This exercise is great for improving your bone health. A lot of age-related bone fractures and falls in women involve the pelvis so that this exercise will target and strengthen your pelvic bone and the surrounding muscles.

To perform this:

1. Stand fully upright in front of a chair as if you are ready to sit and spread your feet shoulder-width apart.
2. Extend your arms in front of you and keep them that way all through the movement.
3. Bend your knees and slowly lower your hips as if you want to sit on the chair, but don't sit. When your butt touches the chair slightly, press into your heels to get back your initial standing position. Repeat that for about 10 to 15 times.

Forearm Plank

This exercise targets your core and shoulders.

Here's how to do it:

1. Get into a push-up position, but with your arms bent at the elbows such that your forearm is supporting your weight.
2. Keep your body off the mat or floor and keep your back straight at all times. Don't raise or drop your hips. This will engage your core. Hold the position for 30 seconds and then drop to your knees. Repeat ten times.

Modified Push-ups

This routine targets your arms, shoulders, and core.

How's how to do it:

1. Kneel on your mat. Place your hands on the mat below your shoulders, and let your knees be behind your hips so that your back is stretched at an angle.
2. Tuck your toes under and tighten your abdominal muscles. Gradually bend your elbows as you lower your chest toward the floor.
3. Push back on your arms to press your chest back to your earlier position. Repeat as many times as is comfortable.

Shoulder Overhead Press

This targets your biceps, shoulders, and back.

To perform this move:

1. With dumbbells in both hands, stand and spread your feet shoulder-width apart.
2. Bring the dumbbells up to the sides of your head and tighten your abdominal muscles.
3. Slowly press the dumbbells up until your arms are straight above your head. Slowly return to the first position. Repeat 10 times. You can also do this exercise while sitting.

Chest Fly

This targets your chest, back, core, and glutes.

To do this:

1. Lie with your back flat on your mat, your knees at an angle close to 90 degrees, and your feet firmly planted on the floor or mat.
2. Hold dumbbells in both hands over your chest. Keep your palms facing each other and gently open your hands away from your chest. Let your upper arms touch the floor without releasing the tension in them.
3. Contract your chest muscles and slowly return the dumbbells to the initial position. Repeat about 10 times.

Single-Leg Hamstring Bridge

This move targets your glutes, quads, and hamstrings.

To do this:

1. Lie flat on your back. Place your feet flat on the floor or mat and spread your bent knees apart.
2. Place your arms flat by your side and lift one leg straight.
3. Contract your glutes as you lift your hips into a bridge position with your arms still in position. Hold for about 2 to 3 seconds and drop your hips to the mat. Repeat about ten times before switching your leg. Do the same again.

Bent-Over Row

This targets your back muscles and spine.

To do this:

1. Hold dumbbells in both hands and stand behind a sturdy object (for example, a chair). Bend forward and rest your head on the chosen object. Relax your neck and slightly bend your knees. With both palms facing each other, pull the dumbbells to touch your ribs. Hold the position for about 2 to 5 seconds and slowly return to the starting position. Repeat 10 to 15 times.

Basic Abs

A distended belly is a common occurrence in older women. This exercise can strengthen and tighten the abdominal muscles bringing them inward toward your spine.

To perform this:

1. Lie on your back with your feet firmly planted on the floor and your knees bent. Relax your upper body, and rest your hands on your thighs.
2. As you exhale, lift yourself upward off the mat or floor. Stop the upward movement when your hands are resting on your knees. Hold the position for about 2 to 5 seconds, and then slowly return to the starting position. Repeat about 20 to 30 times.

Include Exercises in Your Daily Routine

You do not have to hit the gym or plan a time dedicated to working out. You can make exercise part of your daily routine so that you are always getting the proper amount of body movement, whether or not it is time for exercise.

Here are a few tips on how to include exercises into your daily routine.

- Take the stairs (within reason) instead of using the elevator. You don't want to go up a ten-story building using the stairs! If you have a long way to go up or down, take the stairs a couple of flights, and then complete your trip with the elevator.

- When you talk with your family members at home, don't shout from the top floor and bottom floor. Go up or climb down and talk with them.

- Find a sporting activity that you thoroughly enjoy and do it as often as is convenient. When you're doing something you enjoy, you'll hardly think of it as exercise, and you're likely to stay committed.

- If you are at work, instead of sending emails or text messages to coworkers, walk up to them and talk to them face to face.

- If possible, convert your one-on-one meetings to a walking meeting. Hold the meeting while taking a stroll outside.

- Stop a block or two from your destination and walk the rest of the way. Make walking your preferred mode of transportation.

- Take your dog for walks daily. If you don't have a dog, adopt one. It might seem that you are merely walking your dog, but you are exercising your muscles.

- Take brisk walks as often as possible. Remember to put on comfortable shoes when walking briskly. You can bring your walking shoes with you to make it easy for you to change into them.

Staying Safe While Combining Intermittent Fasting and Exercise

Exercising in your fasting window can help you quickly achieve some of the advanced benefits of intermittent fasting. Nevertheless, it is crucial to follow a few general guidelines to keep you safe during the practice.

There are no iron-cast rules about when to exercise, even on fasting days. Observe what works well for you, whether exercising before eating (during the fasting window) or eating before working out (during the eating window). Many women find that exercising on an empty stomach suit their bodies and leaves them feeling energized for the rest of the day. If this is your, set aside time in the morning before your first meal of the day. Some other women find that although they prefer working out on an empty stomach, they feel depleted right after the exercise. In that case, shift your exercise to about 20 to 30 minutes before your first meal of the day. Your body would have rested a bit after your exercise before you break your fast.

If you prefer working out after you break your fast, which is perfectly fine. Eating shortly before your exercise doesn't render your exercises ineffective. Remember that all of our bodies work in different ways. Keep in mind that the goal of working out is to maintain proper body health long into your golden years. You don't need to impress anyone with great abs or biceps, instead impress yourself with how much power you have. Stay committed to your routines, but don't overdo them. If you start feeling weak, that is your cue to take a break.

If you are fasting for longer periods (24 hours or more), you will need to conserve your energy. Consider doing exercises that will not exert too much stress. Take a walk, do some yoga, or any other type of low-intensity exercise.

We could all use someone on our shoulders reminding us to drink more water. And going without food reduces your body's water content even more. Add in higher levels of exertion, and you'll be depleting your water reserves very quickly. So, here is your reminder to always drink adequate amounts of water before, during, and after your workout sessions.

CHAPTER 9: FASTING BEYOND 24 HOURS

36-Hours Fasts

You don't eat for an entire day in a 36-hour fast. For example, if you end dinner on day 1 at 7 pm, your fast will start immediately after; you miss all meals on day 2 and do not eat again until breakfast on day 3 at 7 am. That totals 36 hours of fasting. 36-hour fasts are used in our IDM System, on a three-time-a-week schedule, for patients with type 2 diabetes. We follow this routine until the desired results have been achieved: the patient will quit all medicine for diabetes and has reached the required weight.

After that, we reduce the fasting frequency to a level that allows the patient to keep the hard-won gains but is easier on the patient. How long the three-times-a-week schedule is maintained varies, but in general, the longer diabetes the patient has had, the longer the fasting duration required. Within a couple of weeks, we cannot reverse 20 years of diabetes. But then again, the longer-duration fasting period provides us the power needed in a reasonable time to get good results.

We suggest that blood sugar be tested on a regular basis between two and four times a day, as low blood sugar and high blood sugar are possible. Generally, medicines are reduced on the day of fasting to prevent hypoglycemia, once more, have a dialog with your doctor if you are on medication before doing a fasting regimen. Because changes in medication distress everyone to some extent differently, however, there is the likelihood of too much reduction in medication, which results in high blood sugar. Testing regularly allows you to fine-tune the medication so that you get the same amount you need, no more, no less.

The Warrior Diet

Like the 20:4 plan, the Warrior diet focuses on reducing or stopping all eating completely for 20 hours, followed by enjoying all your daily sustenance within four hours. This is a popular method for people who work out vigorously during the fasting window. There are no restrictions on this plan, and some people may consume a higher percentage of carbs (healthy, natural carbs) and nutrients for their daily meals. This may also include a high level of protein, which helps build muscle tissue. The Warrior diet was made famous by fitness experts and considered one of the best ways to "carb-up" or increase energy during the 4-hour eating window for better physical endurance and performance for the fasting period. This program promotes Paleo and whole, natural (unprocessed) foods, which is ideal if you are familiar with this way of eating and wish to combine this plan with intermittent fasting.

Longer Fasting Periods of 36, 48, 60, and 72 Hours

Experimenting and trying various intermittent fasting plans may lead towards a goal of a multiple-day fast that can exceed a day, sometimes up to two or three consecutive days. Before you attempt a longer fast, start from a 12 or 16-hour fasting window first, then gradually increase your window as you become more comfortable with the process. Jumping into a long-term fast with little or no preparation can lead to exhaustion, fatigue and ultimately lead to breaking the fast prematurely. Ideally, if you plan to fast for more than one day, once you are ready, finding a serene, calm place to unwind and find peace is the best way to reap the rewards of this practice.

In ancient times, a long-term fast would be considered a journey spent in a secluded, calm region, usually in the countryside or in a natural environment where there is little or no interference from the outside world. It's often considered a time of reflection and mediation, which can benefit your well-being in mind and body. Some spas and retreats are ideal for this practice, though camping or taking an extended hike in a wooded or forested area can achieve the same result.

CHAPTER 10: DO NOT REDUCE CALORIES: STIMULATE YOUR METABOLISM

Weight loss has emerged as a billion-dollar industry. It had a market valuation of over 70 billion last year. This is for an industry that didn't even exist a few decades back. The world didn't recognize obesity as a mainstream problem a century ago. Back then, malnutrition was a real problem. However, the circumstances have changed.

Today, obesity is a problem affecting more than 1.9 billion people all over the globe. However, have you ever wondered the reason most people fail to lose weight?

Weight loss is such a big problem because people don't address the correct issue.

Calories Are Not the Cause of Weight Gain

A very big misconception people have in their minds is that a few extra calories are the sole reason for their weight gain. They are wrong.

Burning stored body fat is a much more complex process than you think. Until you don't understand the process, you will keep losing weight and burning body fat.

But, before that, you will have to understand that fat is important for the body, and it fights tooth and nail to conserve this fat.

The Importance of Fat for the Body

Have you ever wondered the reason it is so difficult to burn body fat? It is so difficult because the body values this fat highly, and it tries everything to protect it.

Our body keeps collecting energy from almost every meal that we have and stores it as fat. It protects this fat aggressively because it knows that in a condition of complete energy cut-off, only this fat can help the body survive for the longest.

This is one reason your body wouldn't start burning fat at the first instant of lower energy intake.

However, this is not the only reason your body doesn't begin burning fat immediately. There are two more reasons.

Important Factors for Burning Fat

To burn fat, only the energy deficit is not sufficient ground. Two more things will be required to burn fat. The first is readiness, and the second is the mode.

Let us understand both in detail:

Lack of Readiness-Insulin Resistance

Besides being the facilitator of glucose absorption, insulin is also the key fat-storage hormone. Whatever glucose is left in the bloodstream after the absorption of the cells, insulin stores it in the muscles, liver, and fat tissues.

The glucose in the bloodstream keeps the blood sugar levels high, which can be dangerous for the functioning of the vital organs. It can also affect crucial functions like blood pressure and the elasticity of the muscles. The high blood sugar content can harden the vessels, and they'll become prone to damage. That's the reason it is the job of insulin to lower the blood sugar levels rapidly.

This can be done fastest through absorption by the cells.

However, whatever glucose is left in the bloodstream, insulin starts storing it as glycogen in the muscles. But the muscles can't store a lot of it. As soon as the muscle glycogen stores are full, insulin starts storing glucose as glycogen in the liver.

The liver can store a substantial amount of energy. Your body can run only on the glycogen stored in the liver for almost 36 hours.

However, the glycogen stores of the liver keep filling up regularly, and hence insulin will not get to store a lot there.

The last place to store all the excess glucose is in the adipose tissues. A lot of fat can be stored as subcutaneous fat under your belly, thighs, and hips.

The Detrimental Impact of Insulin Resistance

As you know that insulin is a very important hormone, and it performs several crucial functions. Two key functions are facilitating glucose absorption by the cells and fat storage.

When your cells become insulin resistant, both these functions get affected.

First of all, the cells respond slowly to the insulin signals, and hence your blood sugar levels remain high for longer than required. Due to this, the pancreas starts pumping more insulin as it wants the blood sugar levels to go down. However, more insulin is not solving the problem. More insulin means more exposure to the cells which are already battling overexposure. This escalates the problem further.

This means that the cells wouldn't be in a condition to accept glucose readily, and the blood sugar levels would remain high. To solve this problem, insulin has no other option than to convert glucose into fat rapidly.

Now, insulin is the key fat-storage hormone. As long as there is a high insulin presence in your bloodstream, your body would remain in a fat-storage mode.

Once released by the pancreas, it takes anywhere between 8-12 hours for the insulin levels to go down. Because your body is battling insulin resistance, the insulin levels would be abnormally high because the pancreas keeps pumping more and more insulin.

This also means that your body would remain in a fat storage mode as the insulin levels are unlikely to go down in your body. From your last meal to the next meal, it takes anywhere between 8-12 hours for your insulin levels to go down. If you consume anything between this period, your insulin levels would again shoot up, and your body would stop burning any kind of fat.

Most of us never get that kind of a gap between our meals due to our erratic eating habits. This is one of the chief reasons your body is unlikely to get into a fat-burning mode in normal conditions.

Our erratic habit of eating at short intervals is one of the main culprits of insulin resistance and obesity. You must keep in mind that as long as your body is insulin resistant, it will struggle with burning fat.

Ketosis-The Fat Burning Mode

Another important reason for failure to burn fat is the wrong fuel mode.

Our body can run on two fuel types:

- The glucose fuels
- The fat fuels

You get glucose from the carbs and protein that you consume in your meals. The fat comes from the fat in the meat, fatty fruits, egg yolk, fatty fish, oils, etc.

Your body can easily run on both types of fuel. However, it can't run on both at the same time.

When we are trying to lose weight with the calorie-restriction method or low-calorie diets, we are effectively trying to do just that. We lower the calorie and expect the body to burn fat and glucose at the same time.

This is not going to happen, and it never does. This is the reason most people never burn any real fat despite their best efforts.

The process of burning fat is called ketosis. In this process, your body switches from glucose fuel to fat fuel. Once the body has made the switch, and it is only getting fat fuel to burn, it will easily start burning the body fat as fuel.

However, for this to take place, you will have to stop the intake of glucose fuel. This means that you will have to stop the intake of carbs, and would also have to manage your protein intake strictly as excess protein would also get converted into glucose, ultimately through the process of glucogenesis.

Burning Fat in Reality

If you want to burn fat, you will have to ensure no excess insulin floating in your bloodstream. You will have to keep in mind that no matter what, as long as there is insulin in your bloodstream, your body wouldn't start burning fat as it would remain in a fat storage mode.

This is where intermittent fasting is of special use.

Intermittent fasting is the process of creating prolonged gaps between your meals. With the help of intermittent fasting, you will be able to create longer gaps, so that the insulin levels can go down very long. In such circumstances, your body would be able to burn fat for energy.

Intermittent fasting is also the best way to lower insulin resistance, and hence you can also expect your cells to become more sensitive to insulin signals. This means that there will be less insulin in your bloodstream if your cells respond well to the insulin signals.

Intermittent fasting also creates long gaps of glucose absence. Glucose is a short-lived form of energy. This means that your cells can use glucose rapidly. It provides instant energy, but it doesn't last very long. Hence, if you are more insulin sensitive, your cells would absorb glucose rapidly and use it up fast.

If you consume food again after a short interval, your body will start facing an energy shortage. In the complete absence of glucose, your body can also begin ketosis in which it starts breaking fats to convert them into ketones that can be used as energy.

A fat-rich diet like a ketogenic diet, also called the keto diet, will expedite the process.

The fat that you consume in your diet doesn't get processed in the same way as glucose. It is broken down in the intestines with the help of bile juices released by the gallbladder.

The bile juices help in breaking the fat into smaller parts, and these are then metabolized in the liver.

However, unlike glucose, you don't need insulin to facilitate the absorption of the ketones by the cells. To facilitate the absorption of ketones, the alpha cells in the pancreas releases glucagon. Hence, there is no insulin response at all in your body. This means that your body will be capable of burning the body fat right away if there is any significant need for energy, like heavy exercise.

Therefore, it is with the help of intermittent fasting and a keto diet that you can easily achieve fat-burning much faster and more effectively than any other process.

It is one of the most reliable ways to lose weight rapidly.

You would lose a significant amount of your actual body fat without following a punishing diet or calorie-restriction program. Intermittent fasting is the most scientific way to lose significant weight without compromising your health.

Hormonal Health of Women-The Most Ignored Factor in Weight Loss

One of the most dangerous things that women do while trying to lose weight is that they ignore the importance of their hormonal health.

One of the most significant differences between men and women is the way their bodies treat food.

The body of a man doesn't attach too much significance to food. For men, food is just a way to survive. This is in stark contrast to the way the body of a woman treats food.

For women, food means much more than simple survival; it is connected to their hormonal balance.

From the time a girl hits puberty to the time she reaches menopause, her body is physically always in a readiness mode to bear a child. Bearing a child is a big responsibility. A child in the womb is a big drain on the energy sources in a woman's body. Once a woman conceives a child, her body tries its best to provide nutrition to the child. This was always not possible through conventional mediums in the past.

In the past, women sometimes got food and, most of the time didn't. This can make the survival of the child in the womb difficult. To solve this problem, nature has devised the plan of energy storage inside the body to help the child survive.

This is why women have a comparatively higher body fat ratio than men, and they are also more likely to gain fat rapidly. It is not a weakness they have, but a brilliant plan devised by nature to survive the coming generations.

Food and Female Hormones Are Connected

The hormones in the body are chemical messengers that help in passing on vital information to the brain. Hormones regulate several crucial functions. If you look closely, the life of a woman is completely dominated by these hormones.

The thyroid and pituitary are two very important glands that secrete most of the hormones. They also regulate the behavior of a woman. These glands are also present in men but don't have that profound impact on them simply because they are not going to bear a child.

Women feel a very strong connection with food, and that's why emotional eating, impulsive eating, celebration eating, and all other forms of eating have such strong meanings for women. For women, food is a part of emotional security as it also helps in the regulation and balancing of certain hormones.

Impact of Calorie-Restrictive Diets of Hormonal Balance

Calorie-restrictive diets can harm the hormonal balance in women. It can fill them with a sense of insecurity, void, and unhappiness. Scientific experiments on mice have shown that prolonged calorie-restriction can also lead to the shrinking of female reproductive organs, and they may also lose their ability to reproduce effectively.

Strict diets can also cause irregular periods, and they may also face problems in conception. Women on calorie-restrictive diets can also experience strong and sudden mood swings, and they may also become more temperamental. Anger, frustration, irritation, hopelessness, temptation, and cravings are some of the strong feelings experienced by women on calorie-restrictive diets.

Hormonal Balance is Important

It is very important to understand that hormonal balance is very important. Without the hormonal balance, the overall health of a woman will always remain compromised. This is the problem most women keep facing all their lives.

In the pursuit of weight loss and a slender body, women compromise on their hormonal health and end up paying for problems like PCOS, thyroid, metabolic disorders, and other reproductive issues.

Intermittent Fasting-A Reliable Way to Lose Weight Without Compromising Hormonal Health

Intermittent fasting is a safe way to lose weight as it doesn't force you to compromise your hormonal health. Intermittent fasting doesn't make you starve for food or limit your calorie intake specifically.

It is a process that allows you to eat reasonably. There are no calorie-restrictions. You can eat whatever you feel like as long as you maintain adequate control over quantity.

This eliminates cravings, temptations, and obsessiveness regarding certain food items, and hence your hormones remain in control.

Intermittent fasting is not about what to eat but when to eat. The most important thing in intermittent fasting is to observe abstinence from food for a certain number of hours every day. This period can be efficiently timed to be your sleep time, and hence severe hunger pangs and cravings can easily be avoided.

CHAPTER 11: INTERMITTENT FASTING AND INSULIN

Intermittent fasting can affect women and men differently because of the different hormones present in their bodies.

One notable difference between women and men is that some women have experienced changes to their menstrual cycle when fasting. Women's bodies are more sensitive to small-calorie changes, especially when it comes to a reduction in calorie intake. Since women's bodies are built to conceive and grow babies, their bodies have to be sensitive to changes in the internal environment to a larger degree than the bodies of men.

When women's bodies experience a reduction in calorie intake, they may have trouble experiencing regular menstrual cycles as the body may deem the internal environment less than ideal for a baby to be grown. This effect does not mean that women cannot practice Intermittent Fasting or fasting of any sort, but they must keep this in mind when deciding to try a fasting diet.

Intermittent Fasting and Insulin

Insulin is a hormone that exists in the bodies of both women and men. Intermittent fasting leads to lower levels of the insulin hormone present in the bloodstream during fasting periods.

This effect happens due to the absence of food, specifically sugars, being taken into the body. This process leads to improved use of fat cells for energy, which, over time, increases the effectiveness of insulin, which is one of the main hormones involved in metabolism, as it signals to cells that there has been an intake in sugar, and awakens them to process and store this sugar.

By reducing the sugar, the insulin becomes more sensitive to the body's environment. Over time, this is beneficial for the woman's insulin cells and blood sugar levels practicing intermittent fasting.

Further, when insulin levels are lower, this leads to the release of another hormone called HGH, which also helps in the breakdown and use of stored fat cells for energy, which leads to weight loss.

Another hormone triggered by intermittent fasting is Norepinephrine or Noradrenaline, which becomes released in response to an empty stomach. This hormone encourages the release and the metabolism of fat cells for energy, leading to weight loss and improved health due to a reduction in the increased belly fat often found in women over 50.

The Relationship Between Intermittent Fasting and Fertility

When women are trying to conceive, their bodies are sensitive to the state of the body's internal environment.

This sensitivity is because the body will not allow conception if the environment is not ideal for a healthy fetus's growth.

It is important to ensure that your body is in good shape and has enough nutrients if you are trying to conceive so that the body is confident that it will be able to grow a healthy baby. That being said, some benefits are demonstrated to come about for women following an Intermittent Fasting regime when it comes to fertility, likely because of increased overall health.

Men do not have monthly cycles that they must take into account when fasting, and the hormonal imbalance associated with fasting does not affect them in the same way that it affects women. When you fast, your body produces a heightened amount of the human growth hormone. This hormone benefits men with nearly no negative side-effects, but for women, it has been known to put their delicate hormonal balance off-kilter at times.

The human growth hormone disrupts the female hormone, estrogen if the fasting is not delicately controlled.

I am not saying that women can't fast; it depends on how each woman views their cycles, how regular they are, how active the woman is, and more.

Men can generally do any type of fasting with no harm, under the right health conditions. It is generally recommended for women to fast no more than 16 hours a day to maintain their hormonal balance. This factors into a woman's choice of fasting type. If the woman is very active and used to the occasional skipped period due to vigorous exercise, most fasting types should not be a problem. If a woman is worried about fertility issues, irregular cycles, and more, it may be a better idea to go with the 16/8 or even the 14/10 fasting method. It's all up to preference and personal health concerns, but either way, gender does play a part in your fasting choice.

Intermittent Fasting and Pregnancy

If you are pregnant or breastfeeding, intermittent fasting is a no-go.

There aren't many situations where I would say no to intermittent fasting, but this is a big one. Intermittent fasting is detrimental to a pregnant woman's body because you do not supply the baby with the nutrients it needs during a fasting window. By fasting, you are not allowing your baby to grow and develop at a natural pace fully, and they need all the help they can get.

Additionally, if you breastfeed your infant, intermittent fasting can disrupt milk production and hinder the milk's nutrient content. This effect can lead to dehydration and malnourishment for the baby or a halt in milk production altogether. Either way, intermittent fasting will still be there once the baby grows up and stops requiring your body's nutritional assistance. If the milk is made in a healthy body, it will be healthy milk and help the baby be healthy.

If you give birth and then immediately go on a strict diet to try to lose your baby weight, this is not a good idea and will not lead to healthy milk being produced.

Doing the act of breastfeeding each day causes you to burn calories, and thus, you will still need to consume more calories than you did before getting pregnant, even though your baby is no longer in your womb. While breastfeeding, don't go on any diet, and don't begin to watch what you eat unless it is to ensure you are eating enough. You want to have as many nutrients and calories as your baby needs, so listen to your hunger and follow what it tells you.

Specific Intermittent Fasting Methods for Women Who Are Trying to Conceive

While pregnant or breastfeeding women should avoid intermittent fasting and instead stick to a well-rounded, whole food diet, women trying to conceive can still use this dieting method, with some considerations.

- **Fast for Only 14 Hours or Less**

Over the years, nutritionists have theorized that though you do not go into the highest ketosis level until 16 hours of fasting, the 14-hours mark may be better for women. You still go into ketosis at hour fourteen, so it is still beneficial for weight loss, but as you do not reach a heightened ketosis level, the side effects aren't as prominent either. Nutritionists believe that this is a good middle-ground for women because it has been hypothesized that higher ketosis levels may disrupt a woman's hormones and thus their menstrual cycles. For this reason, women who are trying to conceive should avoid methods of intermittent fasting that involve a fasting window of more than 14 hours, such as the 16/8 or the 24 hours fast. Instead, it is best to stick to a 14/10 or a 12 hour fast. A woman's hormones must be regulated and normal if she hopes to conceive.

- **Use Exercise as Your Primary means Of Autophagy Induction**

As I mentioned earlier in this book, women may experience different effects when they attempt intermittent fasting than men. For this reason, women may opt to use exercise as the main method of autophagy induction. This point is especially important if they are trying to conceive or if they have experienced irregularities with their menstrual cycle in the past. They can also use intermittent fasting and exercise combined, with shorter fasting periods such as 12 and 12, coupled with an aerobic exercise routine.

Poly-Cystic Ovarian Syndrome (PCOS)

PCOS or Polycystic Ovarian Syndrome is something that many women suffer from. This disease leads women's ovaries to develop cysts, leading to very painful periods, weight gain, and infertility. For women who suffer from Polycystic Ovarian Syndrome, it can be very hard to lose weight. By following intermittent fasting, however, women with Polycystic Ovarian Syndrome have been able to lose weight while also having relief from many of the other symptoms associated with it. It has been shown that a diet high in carbohydrates can negatively affect Polycystic Ovarian Syndrome and can exacerbate symptoms. By following an intermittent fasting regime, which is also lower in carbohydrates, women's bodies showed improvement in their general health, reduced the symptoms of this disease (including leading to weight loss), and helped mitigate the progression of the disease.

CHAPTER 12: MENOPAUSE AND INTERMITTENT FASTING

The Menstrual Cycle

When fasting, some women have experienced changes in their menstrual cycle. The bodies of women are more sensitive to small-calorie changes, especially when it comes to a reduction in calorie intake. Since the bodies of women are built to conceive and grow babies, their bodies have to be sensitive to changes in the internal environment to a larger degree than the bodies of men. When the bodies of women experience a reduction in calorie intake, they may have trouble experiencing regular menstrual cycles as the body may deem the internal environment less than ideal for a baby to be grown. This is not to say that women cannot practice Intermittent fasting or fasting of any sort, but that they must keep this in mind when deciding to try a fasting diet.

Intermittent Fasting and Menopause

Intermittent fasting in women has been shown to lead to the release of hormones that, in turn, lead to the release of bone minerals such as phosphate and calcium, and the release of these bone minerals leads to increase bone density and strength, which is especially beneficial in women who are over 50, as the risk of developing osteoporosis is very high. Therefore, inducing autophagy in the body leads to a reduction in the risk of developing osteoporosis in women over 50, and can even lead to improvements in women who have already been diagnosed with it.

When it comes to menopause, many things in your body can feel like they are out of your control. Menopause can lead to weight gain, depression, anxiety, and increased risk of heart disease, among others. It will also lead to changes in the hormones and the metabolism of the women that are in menopause, as well as a reduction in the body's sensitivity to insulin.

Because of all of these side-effects that come with menopause, intermittent fasting has been tested as a method for reducing those side-effects and has shown to be useful in improving them. Intermittent fasting has proven to be a good choice for improving the symptoms of menopause, such as the pesky weight gain that many women experience, reducing the risk of heart disease, reducing depression, as well as improved cognitive functioning. Therefore, not only can intermittent fasting improve the way you feel about your body and yourself in general during this time of transition, but it can also make you live a longer and healthier life.

CHAPTER 13: THE 7 SECRETS TO LOSE WEIGHT

1. Chew Slowly and Rest the Fork After Each Mouthful

When you chew slowly, you are able to discern the different taste sensations that each mouthful brings to your palate. This allows you to get all the nutrients and vitamins from the food served into your body system. It also delays how quickly you feel full, which keeps you from overeating. Chewing food properly helps you to digest the food that you eat correctly, and ensure that all nutrients are absorbed in the correct manner. It also helps to reduce the calories in your stomach faster, which is healthy to lose weight.

2. Eat More Proteins than Carbohydrates

Proteins are the building blocks of muscles and other organs, and they are the single most important nutrients that the body needs. Proteins are comprised of amino acids; which include essential amino acids required for growth and repair as well as several non-essential ones. You need to get a high percentage of your daily calories from proteins in order to remain healthy.

3. Eat a Lot of Dietary Fiber; Including Fruits and Vegetables

Dietary fiber improves the digestive process and flow of food through your body. Most fruits are rich in dietary fiber, but it is recommended that you eat more vegetables because they help the digestive system to work better while providing essential vitamins, minerals, and other nutrients into the body.

4. Eat in Small Dishes and Bowls

Eating in small dishes makes each meal seem more satisfying, and the space in your stomach remains full for longer. This keeps you from overeating. Eating food as if it is going out of style also ensures that you derive the maximum reward for your money when buying food from restaurants.

5. Drink Only Water, Tea, and Coffee Eliminating Fizzy Drinks

A study conducted at the University of Wisconsin-Madison has proven that drinking as little as 4.5 fluid ounces of soda causes weight gain, especially among teenagers. If you go to a restaurant and order a soft drink, then you are likely to eat more than you should. By avoiding energy drinks, caffeinated drinks, and fizzy drinks, you will not only save money but also ensure that your diet is healthy to ensure good health and wellbeing.

Water keeps the body hydrated; it helps maintain normal body temperature by removing unwanted heat from the body. Water promotes blood circulation, which aids in removing toxins from the body and helps to avoid diseases such as kidney stones.

6. Eat Without Distractions (No TV, No Cell Phone)

You should attempt to eat without watching TV or talking on the cell phone. By doing this, you will have a clear mind and be able to concentrate on your meal. This will prevent you from eating more than you should, and it will also reduce compulsive eating later on.

7. Sleep At Least 8 Hours per Night

To lose weight, you should sleep 8 hours each night. During sleep, the body releases certain chemicals that help the digestive process and also helps you to burn fat more efficiently. Having proper sleep also restores the body and mind, and boosts your energy levels, which is essential for burning fat.

CONCLUSION

Thank you for purchasing this book, "Intermittent Fasting for Women Over 50".

For women over 50s, dieting is not an option; it's a necessity. By employing intermittent fasting as part of their daily routine, you will be able to shed pounds and maintain a healthier lifestyle for years to come!

Here are some tips for you to be able to succeed in intermittent fasting, especially now that you are in your 50s already:

1. Eat only when you are hungry.

2. Drink plenty of water to keep your metabolism high.

3. If you are going to more than 48 hours without food, ensure that you drink sufficient amounts of water (about half your body weight in ounces), and use the restroom frequently to make sure that you do not get dehydrated while fasting.

4. Do not exercise while fasting, as this will just increase your hunger pangs and make it harder for you to fast. Afterward, you can work out as desired since exercise helps with weight loss on a number of levels, including boosting the metabolic rate and burning calories even when at rest!

5. Do not start intermittent fasting without the supervision of your doctor. That being said, once you are both on the same page, intermittent fasting is very safe and super healthy.

6. Be on the lookout for hunger pangs! Hunger pangs can be eased by eating some heart-healthy olives or nuts (consult with your doctor first) or sipping on some black coffee to stimulate the release of leptin (a hormone that suppresses appetite).

7. Keep yourself busy and do not think about food! This is easier said than done, I know, but it will keep your mind off eating so much.

Since intermittent fasting is not limiting in what you can eat, there is a wide variety to choose from. All you have to keep in mind is the number of calories you are consuming per meal. Meals that have low carbohydrate content are ideal because they, in turn, have low caloric content as well. Having more lean meats, fruits, and vegetables is ideal together with grains too.

Learn as many recipes as possible, and prepare them for yourself in order to better manage the ingredients being used. You can even do a meal prep whereby you take one day to prepare the meals you wish to eat during the coming week. This means even when you are too busy or too tired to cook, all you have to do is get your prepped meal, warm it, and enjoy a healthy meal. One reason to go for fast food is that it is readily available. Preparing your meals in advance can help you cover this.

Reaching the end of our book brings with us mixed emotions and happiness at how much knowledge we have imparted on you, sadness because this means our conversations are coming to an end.

Intermittent Fasting can be the key to your success in achieving your goals and keeping your body healthy. That is why we encourage you to try it out for yourself and see the benefits that may await you! Now go on, start this journey as soon as possible with this guide! Good luck!

Thank you.